How To Get Rid Of Hemorrhoids

329 Great Tips To Prevent And Cure Hemorrhoids And Piles

ADAM COLTON

Published by BizMove
www.bizmove.com

ISBN: 1978448961
ISBN- 978-1978448964

Table of Contents

1. Hemorrhoids Fact Sheet

What are hemorrhoids?

Hemorrhoids, also called piles, are swollen and inflamed veins around your anus or in your lower rectum.

The two types of hemorrhoids are

- external hemorrhoids, which form under the skin around the anus
- internal hemorrhoids, which form in the lining of the anus and lower rectum

The two types of hemorrhoids are external and internal.

How common are hemorrhoids?

Hemorrhoids are common in both men and women[1] and affect about 1 in 20 Americans.[2] About half of adults older than age 50 have hemorrhoids.[2]

Who is more likely to get hemorrhoids?

You are more likely to get hemorrhoids if you

- strain during bowel movements
- sit on the toilet for long periods of time
- have chronic constipation or diarrhea
- eat foods that are low in fiber
- are older than age 50
- are pregnant
- often lift heavy objects

What are the complications of hemorrhoids?

Complications of hemorrhoids can include the following:

- blood clots in an external hemorrhoid
- skin tags—extra skin left behind when a blood clot in an external hemorrhoid dissolves
- infection of a sore on an external hemorrhoid
- strangulated hemorrhoid—when the muscles around your anus cut off the blood supply to an internal hemorrhoid that has fallen through your anal opening
- anemia

What are the symptoms of hemorrhoids?

The symptoms of hemorrhoids depend on the type you have.

If you have external hemorrhoids, you may have

- anal itching

- one or more hard, tender lumps near your anus
- anal ache or pain, especially when sitting

Too much straining, rubbing, or cleaning around your anus may make your symptoms worse. For many people, the symptoms of external hemorrhoids go away within a few days.

If you have internal hemorrhoids, you may have

- bleeding from your rectum—bright red blood on stool, on toilet paper, or in the toilet bowl after a bowel movement
- a hemorrhoid that has fallen through your anal opening, called prolapse

Internal hemorrhoids that are not prolapsed most often are not painful. Prolapsed internal hemorrhoids may cause pain and discomfort.

Although hemorrhoids are the most common cause of anal symptoms, not every anal symptom is caused by a hemorrhoid. Some hemorrhoid symptoms are similar to those of other digestive tract problems. For example, bleeding from your rectum may be a sign of bowel diseases such as Crohn's disease, ulcerative colitis, or cancer of the colon or rectum .

When should I seek a doctor's help?

You should seek a doctor's help if you

- still have symptoms after 1 week of at-home treatment
- have bleeding from your rectum

What causes hemorrhoids?

The causes of hemorrhoids include

- straining during bowel movements
- sitting on the toilet for long periods of time
- chronic constipation or diarrhea
- a low-fiber diet
- weakening of the supporting tissues in your anus and rectum that happens with aging
- pregnancy
- often lifting heavy objects

How are hemorrhoids diagnosed?

Your doctor can often diagnose hemorrhoids based on your medical history and a physical exam. He or she can diagnose external hemorrhoids by checking the area around your anus. To diagnose internal hemorrhoids, your doctor will perform a digital rectal exam and may perform procedures to look inside your anus and rectum.

Medical history

Your doctor will ask you to provide your medical history and describe your symptoms. He or she will ask you about your eating habits, toilet habits, enema and laxative use, and current medical conditions.

Your doctor will ask you to provide your medical history and describe your symptoms.

Physical exam

Your doctor will check the area around your anus for

- lumps or swelling
- internal hemorrhoids that have fallen through your anal opening, called prolapse
- external hemorrhoids with a blood clot in a vein
- leakage of stool or mucus
- skin irritation
- skin tags—extra skin that is left behind when a blood clot in an external hemorrhoid dissolves
- anal fissures—a small tear in the anus that may cause itching, pain, or bleeding

Your doctor will perform a digital rectal exam to

- check the tone of the muscles in your anus

- check for tenderness, blood, internal hemorrhoids, and lumps or masses

Procedures

Your doctor may use the following procedures to diagnose internal hemorrhoids:

- **Anoscopy.** For an anoscopy, your doctor uses an anoscope to view the lining of your anus and lower rectum. Your doctor will carefully examine the tissues lining your anus and lower rectum to look for signs of lower digestive tract problems and bowel disease. Your doctor performs an anoscopy during an office visit or at an outpatient center. Most patients do not need anesthesia .

- **Rigid proctosigmoidoscopy.** Rigid proctosigmoidoscopy is similar to anoscopy, except that your doctor uses an instrument called a proctoscope to view the lining of your rectum and lower colon. Your doctor will carefully examine the tissues lining your rectum and lower colon to look for signs of lower digestive tract problems and bowel disease. Your doctor performs this procedure during an office visit or at an outpatient center or a hospital. Most patients do not need anesthesia.

Your doctor may diagnose internal hemorrhoids while performing procedures for other digestive tract problems or during routine examination of your rectum and colon. These procedures include colonoscopy and flexible sigmoidoscopy.

How can I treat my hemorrhoids?

You can most often treat your hemorrhoids at home by

- eating foods that are high in fiber
- taking a stool softener or a fiber supplement such as psyllium (Metamucil) or methylcellulose (Citrucel)
- drinking water or other nonalcoholic liquids each day as recommended by your health care professional
- not straining during bowel movements
- not sitting on the toilet for long periods of time
- taking over-the-counter pain relievers such as acetaminophen , ibuprofen , naproxen , or aspirin
- sitting in a tub of warm water, called a sitz bath, several times a day to help relieve pain

Applying over-the-counter hemorrhoid creams or ointments or using suppositories—a medicine you insert into your rectum—may relieve mild pain, swelling, and itching of external hemorrhoids. Most often, doctors recommend using over-the-counter products for 1 week. You should follow up with your doctor if the products

- do not relieve your symptoms after 1 week
- cause side effects such dry skin around your anus or a rash

Most prolapsed internal hemorrhoids go away without at-home treatment. However, severely prolapsed or bleeding internal hemorrhoids may need medical treatment.

How do doctors treat hemorrhoids?

Doctors treat hemorrhoids with procedures during an office visit or in an outpatient center or a hospital.

Office treatments include the following:

- **Rubber band ligation.** Rubber band ligation is a procedure that doctors use to treat bleeding or prolapsing internal hemorrhoids. A doctor places a special rubber band around the base of the hemorrhoid. The band cuts off the blood supply. The banded part of the hemorrhoid shrivels and falls off, most often within a week. Scar tissue forms in the remaining part of the hemorrhoid, often shrinking the hemorrhoid. Only a doctor should perform this procedure—you should never try this treatment yourself.

- **Sclerotherapy.** A doctor injects a solution into an internal hemorrhoid, which causes scar tissue to form. The scar tissue cuts off the blood supply, often shrinking the hemorrhoid.
- **Infrared photocoagulation.** A doctor uses a tool that directs infrared light at an internal hemorrhoid. Heat created by the infrared light causes scar tissue to form, which cuts off the blood supply, often shrinking the hemorrhoid.
- **Electrocoagulation.** A doctor uses a tool that sends an electric current into an internal hemorrhoid. The electric current causes scar tissue to form, which cuts off the blood supply, often shrinking the hemorrhoid.

Outpatient center or hospital treatments include the following:

- **Hemorrhoidectomy.** A doctor, most often a surgeon, may perform a hemorrhoidectomy to remove large external hemorrhoids and prolapsing internal hemorrhoids that do not respond to other treatments. Your doctor will give you anesthesia for this treatment.
- **Hemorrhoid stapling.** A doctor, most often a surgeon, may use a special stapling tool to remove internal hemorrhoid tissue and pull a prolapsing internal hemorrhoid back into the

anus. Your doctor will give you anesthesia for this treatment.

Sometimes complications of hemorrhoids also require treatment.

Seek care right away

You should seek medical care right away if you have severe anal pain and bleeding from your rectum, particularly with discomfort or pain in your abdomen, diarrhea, or fever.

How can I prevent hemorrhoids?

You can help prevent hemorrhoids by

- eating foods that are high in fiber
- drinking water or other nonalcoholic liquids each day as recommended by your health care professional
- not straining during bowel movements
- not sitting on the toilet for long periods of time
- avoiding regular heavy lifting

What should I eat if I have hemorrhoids?

Your doctor may recommend that you eat more foods that are high in fiber. Eating foods that are high in fiber can make stools softer and easier to pass and can help treat and prevent hemorrhoids.

Drinking water and other liquids, such as fruit juices and clear soups, can help the fiber in your diet work better. Ask your doctor about how much you should drink each day based on your health and activity level and where you live.

The Dietary Guidelines for Americans recommends a dietary fiber intake of 14 grams per 1,000 calories consumed. For example, for a 2,000-calorie diet, the fiber recommendation is 28 grams per day.

What should I avoid eating if I have hemorrhoids?

If your hemorrhoids are caused by chronic constipation, try not to eat too many foods with little or no fiber, such as

- cheese
- chips
- fast food
- ice cream
- meat
- prepared foods, such as some frozen and snack foods
- processed foods, such as hot dogs and some microwavable dinners

2. 329 Great Tips To Prevent And Cure Hemorrhoids And Piles

Hemorrhoids can be a painful and somewhat embarrassing medical problem for any sufferer. You can do something about your discomfort and relieve yourself from this common condition. You deserve the comfort and peace of mind that comes from taking charge of your situation and finding solutions to your hemorrhoid distress. The following tips will help you in this matter.

1. Constipation can contribute to the development of hemorrhoids or make them worse if you currently have them. Consume a diet rich in high-fiber foods or take a fiber supplement every day. Drink plenty of water along with the extra fiber as this will help your stool to become softer and easier to pass.

2. In order to soften your food to help with hemorrhoids, try to consume foods that are high in fiber. Some fruits that are high in fiber are watermelon, grapes, and papaya. Okra, kangkong, and cabbage are veggies that are high in fiber. Be

sure that you consume eight to ten glasses of water each day.

3. Are you aware there are many items in your kitchen that can lessen the symptoms of hemorrhoids? You can create your own ice pack for instance. Ice packs can numb the pain and reduce swelling. If you place ice packs on you hemorrhoids, they can cut down on the amount of swelling.

4. If you are looking for natural relief from your hemorrhoids, eating certain foods can help. To reduce bleeding, try alfalfa, blackstrap molasses, flax seeds, sweet potatoes and lima beans. In order to prevent an iron deficiency from loss of blood, try eating chicken or beef liver, prunes, spinach, raisins, tuna, kelp, baked potatoes and sunflower seeds.

5. Beans are very important to help eliminate hemorrhoids. When you consume beans, you will maximize the quality of your bowel movements, which can help with the irritation that you may get from hemorrhoids. Try to eat a least one meal during the day with beans to help improve your condition.

6. People who have colon or digestive tract problems usually also suffer from hemorrhoids. The frequent diarrhea and constipation associated with these

problems can cause hemorrhoids. In order to decrease constipation, you need to eat foods that are rich in fibers. Adding fiber-rich vegetables, fruits and whole grains to your dietary intake can offer relief to colon or digestive tract problems and reduce the chances of developing hemorrhoids.

7. If you believe that you have hemorrhoids that aren't going away with over the counter remedies, seek the advice of a doctor. Many treatments are now able to be performed in the office with minimal discomfort or needed follow up care. You can try an over the counter remedy first, but always follow up with your doctor.

8. In the morning, one of the best drinks that you can have is vegetable juice for your hemorrhoids. Vegetable juice will give you the nutrients that you need to improve blood circulation in your body and can reduce your level of toxins. Drink 16-20 ounces of vegetable juice to start your morning off right.

9. To prevent hemorrhoids make sure you eat a high-fiber diet and drink plenty of water. Unnecessary strain when making a bowel movement is one of the leading causes of hemorrhoids. Including high-fiber foods in your diet will allow everything to pass along smoothly and prevent irritation to the

intestinal walls and anus. Foods that are high in fiber include bran cereals, fruits and vegetables.

10.   Don't depend solely on some over the counter drugs such as laxatives. These are not a cure for constipation, and are meant to just be taken every once in awhile. Many times these types of drugs will help for one bowel movement, and then will end up leaving you more constipated after that.

11.   Use moist toilet tissue or non-alcohol wipes when cleaning yourself on the toilet. Dry paper equates to rough paper no matter the softness of the tissue. The paper can cause bleeding from the hemorrhoids and should be avoided if possible. If you have access to a bidet you can use this as an alternative for paper.

12.   Keep your body hydrated. If your body does not have enough water to function properly, it will remove it from other sources, such as your stools. This has the unfortunate effect of hardening the stool, which then leads to pain and strain during bowel movements. Drink at least eight glasses of water a day. This will help to prevent hemorrhoids. If you already have hemorrhoids, evacuation will go much smoother.

13.   Lower the amount of salt that you take in. Too much salt in your diet can be dehydrating, which is the leading cause of constipation and hemorrhoids. Making choices that have less salt, and upping your fluid intake can decrease any chances that you have issues with using the restroom.

14.   You can soothe your painful, itchy, inflamed hemorrhoids with plain water! Cold water compresses can help as well as a sitz bath you can find at most any pharmacy. It fits over the toilet seat and you can fill it with warm water for a soothing effect. sit on the sitz bath for about 10 minutes for best effects.

15.   Be very careful if you are taking laxatives to soften your stools. These can actually be addictive and sometimes end up causing a lot more harm than good. You should never opt for a laxative unless you are really constipated. For anything else, go with products like natural fiber or stool softener. Consider linseed or psyllium husks.

16.   Eating too much salt can cause you to retain a lot of water and thus increase your odds of swelling, including that hemorrhoid! Your veins can swell with too much salt and that pain and discomfort will return. Reduce your salt to reduce the size and pain associated with hemorrhoids.

17.   An all natural astringent like witch hazel costs only two or three dollars and is available at nearly every pharmacy and grocery store. Soak a cotton ball in the witch hazel, then apply it directly to the surface and surrounding area of your external hemorrhoid. Witch hazel causes the blood vessels to temporarily shrink, which reduces the size and discomfort of the hemorrhoid.

18.   Natural remedies offer great relief from hemorrhoid pain and help you to save money. Many people swear by sitz baths to relieve pain, particularly if you have had a strenuous bowel movement. Hemorrhoids can be quite itchy, but you want to avoid scratching because this will just aggravate the area more. Instead, you can put some witch hazel on a cotton pad and put it on the affected area. Drink at least eight cups of water each day, and eat plenty of fiber. This will prevent excessive straining during a bowel movement.

19.   Your job or lifestyle may have an effect on your hemorrhoid symptoms. If you have a desk job or spend a lot of time sitting while you're at home, make sure to give yourself some relief by walking around for a few minutes every hour. This takes the direct pressure off your hemorrhoids. Also, if your job involves a lot of heavy lifting, try to exhale as

you bear the brunt of the load. Holding your breath exerts pressure on the hemorrhoids and may cause them to become more painful.

20.   Use proper lifting techniques with heavy objects. The strain you put on your body with lifting is equivalent to the stress of straining in the bathroom. This can not only affect other areas of your body, but strain your anus as well. If you can avoid lifting heavy objects all together you will keep the strain to a minimum.

21.   A great way to keep your hemorrhoid problems at bay is to eat foods that are high in fiber. This helps by softening your stool and making it pass easier. Along with the fiber, eat lots of fruits like grapes, watermelon, and papaya, as well as vegetables which are high in fiber like okra and cabbage.

22.   Lay on your side to alleviate pressure. Sitting upright or laying on your back may inadvertently cause more pressure to the rectal area, so relieve that pressure by laying and sleeping on your side. This is especially true for hemorrhoids caused by pregnancy, and the expanding uterus is pulled down toward the rectal area, causing more pressure.

23.   For hemorrhoids that seem to be protruding outside your body, try to gently nudge them back where they belong. Make sure your hands are clean to avoid infections. After pushing the hemorrhoids back inside your body, you should make an appointment with a doctor so that they can be sure that everything is okay.

24.   If your hemorrhoids are causing an extreme amount of itching, you may want to continue taking a warm bath. Be sure to fill the tub with warm water. The warmth of the water will help relieve the itchiness while also cleaning away and dirt of bacteria that may be in the area.

25.   Be sure to stay away from alcohol if you want to avoid developing hemorrhoids. Too much alcohol, even wine, can cause your to become dehydrated. Dehydration is one of the many causes of hemorrhoids. Also, alcohol causes constipation, which causes hemorrhoids because you have to push your stools out too hard.

26.   Make sure to keep your anal area clean in order to prevent hemorrhoids. One of the causes of hemorrhoids is lack of hygiene. Be sure to wipe well after a bowel movement. Also, when you are in the shower be sure to clean your anal area, but do not rub too hard.

27.   To help clear up your hemorrhoids, the first step is to relieve the symptoms. Constipation is a common cause of hemorrhoids, so make sure that your diet is healthy and rich in fiber. Eat lots of fruits and vegetables. Keep the anal area clean to help reduce the painful swelling and itching.

28.   A product like petroleum jelly can work wonders for hemorrhoid flare-ups or even if you have hemorrhoids that aren't flaring up on you. The jelly not only instantly soothes the pain, but it also creates a lubricant that can allow waste to slide past the vein without irritating your hemorrhoid.

29.   If you cannot find any special type of toilet paper out there that's easier on your anus, you should try making sure you only wipe your rear with toilet paper that is wet. This will certainly help to eliminate the friction and create a softer barrier between the paper and the swollen veins in your rectum.

30.   Try using witch hazel if you have hemorrhoids. This product can be found in any drug store or pharmacy. Apply conservative amounts of witch hazel to the hemorrhoids, and their astringent properties will aid in relieving swelling and bleeding.

31.   Some everyday products work wonders for hemorrhoids, and using something as simple and affordable as apple cider vinegar can help you to heal hemorrhoids. The acid in the vinegar will help you in the digestion of your food, and this will ultimately create smaller, looser bowel movements that will not cause your veins to become irritated.

32.   A great tip for your painful hemorrhoids is to make sure that no matter what condition you are in, do not strain when going to the bathroom. Let it happen naturally and never try to force yourself because if you do you are certain to cause a hemorrhoid or hurt an existing one.

33.   Avoid hemorrhoids by eating a high-fiber diet. Fiber, especially soluble fiber, can help keep things moving without irritating your gastrointestinal tract. Examples of foods that are high in fiber, include cabbage, watermelon, and grapes. Increase your fiber intake slowly, to avoid shocking your system and backing things up even worse.

34.   There is a special method available for cleaning just the affected part of your body during this affliction. This is known as a sitz bath and it is a way to cleanse just the rectum and buttocks without the necessity of an entire shower several times a day. This can help greatly.

35.　　If you find that you are in constant pain from hemorrhoids and you are overweight, you may want to consider starting a serious diet and fitness routine. If you can lose some weight, you will eliminate some of the pressure that the extra weight is putting on the veins that are in the anus, which causes the hemorrhoids.

36.　　To prevent the development of hemorrhoids, avoid becoming constipated. Constipation can lead to straining during bowel movements, which is one of the primary causes of hemorrhoids. Eating plenty of fiber, drinking plenty of water and taking a stool softener as needed can all prevent constipation, as can daily exercise.

37.　　Use some witch hazel on a cotton ball to relieve pain and to work to get rid of your hemorrhoids. The witch hazel will work to contract blood vessels and reduce the swelling and stop the bleeding, providing instant pain relief. For an even better result, put the witch hazel on ice before you apply. You will feel instant pain relief from your hemorrhoids.

38.　　Stay clean! Take care of your hemorrhoids! When you go to the restroom, make sure you clean the area thoroughly, taking care not to irritate it. If your bottom is not clean, bacteria can make its way into your hemorrhoids, and cause inflammation or even an abscess. To prevent these painful occurrences, make sure you wash well and prevent irritation!

39.	The best way to avoid the pain of hemorrhoids is to keep the anus and the area surrounding the anus meticulously clean. This will help keep the hemorrhoids from becoming infected and ease any pain. If the hemorrhoids have a bacterial infection, this can lead to an abscess in the area which is very unhealthy and painful.

40.	If you have problems with hemorrhoids, you may find that constipation makes the condition worse. Most Americans don't eat enough fiber. Getting the right amount, approximately 20-40 grams per day, can soften stools and lessen the effect of constipation on hemorrhoids. Foods like fruits, whole-grain cereals and other fiber-rich foods are important for any diet.

41.	Try to avoid eating foods that give you diarrhea if you have a hemorrhoid. There's a common misconception out there that having liquid stools is actually good because it will not cause flare-ups. This is wrong simply because the constant wiping associated with frequent bowel movements will cause irritation.

42.   Purchasing a softer toilet paper is a great way to make sure that you do not cause your hemorrhoids to swell up and become painful. It may cost a little more, but you can find toilet paper with aloe and other lotions and/or oils. These are softer and gentler on your swollen veins.

43.   Try not to take laxative medications if you can help it. While they will help you use the restroom after you take them, they cause further constipation later on. This will only exacerbate your discomfort and frustration. Find other ways to treat your hemorrhoids; consider changing your diet or taking supplements.

44.   Eating corn is actually a great way in which you can help to reduce the pain and swelling of your hemorrhoids. As you may have noticed before, corn doesn't exactly break down well in your stomach. What this means for you is that stools containing corn pass through easier with a lot less friction.

45.   Be gentle on those painful hemorrhoids by easing up on the extremely hot foods. This may be self-explanatory if you have experienced it yourself, but many times the spicy food that you consume

ends up irritating your current hemorrhoids, or or even causing excruciating pain.

46.   Are you looking for natural ways to alleviate the pain, itching and swelling of hemorrhoids? Here is a tip that may help! For pain and swelling, aloe vera can offer quick relief. You can try an aloe vera gel, or if you have access to an aloe vera plant, take the outer layer off of a leaf and place the leaf around the anal area. This technique can soothe pain and itching as well as inflammation!

47.   A great tip for your painful hemorrhoids is to stay away from lifting heavy items as much as you can. This is beneficial advice because you actually end up using the same types of muscles that you would use when straining on the toilet and this can lead to increased pain.

48.   Hemorrhoids can have many irritating and painful symptoms. These include pain, itching, inflammation and bleeding. For some quick relief, a good home remedy is apple cider vinegar. Dip a cotton swab in the vinegar and dab it gently over the inflamed hemorrhoids. Do this twice a day for soothing relief.

49.   If you have hemorrhoids try increasing your physical activity daily. Sitting for long periods of

time can increase your likelihood of getting hemorrhoids and walking around can decrease the pain and allow them to heal themselves faster. Sitting stretches the area out while moving around allows the area to relax.

50.   Over the counter creams and ointments are one of the more affordable options for relief from the pain and discomfort of hemorrhoids. Look for soothing ingredients to treat different symptoms. Ingredients like hydrocortisone will reduce itching and swelling, while local anesthetics will provide effective, but temporary relief from pain and soreness.

51.   Avoid hemorrhoids by eating a high-fiber diet. Fiber, especially soluble fiber, can help keep things moving without irritating your gastrointestinal tract. Examples of foods that are high in fiber, include cabbage, watermelon, and grapes. Increase your fiber intake slowly, to avoid shocking your system and backing things up even worse.

52.   If you are struggling with hemorrhoids, it could be because you are overweight. When you are overweight the pressure increases in your waist and abdominal area. This could cause you to have increases pressure in the veins of the anus. You can fix this problem by losing some weight which will

reduce the pressure. In addition, if you eat less you will likely pass smaller stools, and you will need to do so less often too.

53.   A wonderful and lesser-known remedy for treating hemorrhoids is emu oil. Emu oil is made from the fat of the emu, a large bird native to Australia. This amazing oil is anti-bacterial and anti-inflammatory. It promotes healing and thickens thinning skin, making it an excellent choice for the treatment of hemorrhoids.

54.   To maximize the way that you feel during the day and reduce your hemorrhoids, try to incorporate acai berries into your diet. These berries are very rich in antioxidants and can help break down the toxins in your body. This will help your hemorrhoids disappear and improve the way that you feel.

55.   If you have hemorrhoids and find that your problem hasn't taken care of itself after a couple of weeks or the problem seems to be getting worse quickly than you should go to a professional immediately. Probably you will have no major problems but they will be able to tell you exactly what is going on.

56.   One of the easiest home treatments to aid in the healing, from the painful burning and itching of hemorrhoids, is a sitz bath. A good recipe for a sitz bath is witch hazel. Fill your tub with warm water and add at least one cup of witch hazel to your water. Sit in this warm mixture for 10-15 minutes, at least three times per day. Within three to four days, your hemorrhoids will be gone.

57.   If you are planning on going out with your friends, try to avoid alcohol at all costs. It is very important to stay hydrated when you have hemorrhoids, as alcohol will just serve to dehydrate you even further. Stick to water or refrain from drinking when you are going out.

58.   Changing your diet is going to help you avoid getting more hemorrhoids. If you start consuming different types of fresh fruits and vegetables you are going to loosen your stool and make it easier to pass. This will help prevent more hemorrhoids from forming from harsh bowel movements.

59.   You should drink eight eight-ounce glasses of water each day to help you to prevent hemorrhoids. Also, water is needed to soften your stool which will also reduce the pain related to hemorrhoids. Limiting alcohol and caffeine intake can also work in your favor, as they both promote loss of water

from your body. Keep yourself hydrated, drink enough water.

60.   Eat as much high-fiber foods as you can. This will help to soften your stool and help prevent hemorrhoids from forming. Most fruit, like grapes, watermelon and papaya, has a lot of fiber in it. Any kind of roughage will also be helpful. You can take fiber pills, as well, to aid in the process.

61.   Use some witch hazel on a cotton ball to relieve pain and to work to get rid of your hemorrhoids. The witch hazel will work to contract blood vessels and reduce the swelling and stop the bleeding, providing instant pain relief. For an even better result, put the witch hazel on ice before you apply. You will feel instant pain relief from your hemorrhoids.

62.   To reduce the chances of developing hemorrhoids, maintain a healthy weight. Being overweight puts excessive pressure on the pelvic region and the pelvic veins. The best way to maintain a healthy weight and prevent hemorrhoids, is to get plenty of exercise and eat a well balanced diet that is high in fiber.

63.   A great way to keep your hemorrhoid problems at bay is to eat foods that are high in fiber. This

helps by softening your stool and making it pass easier. Along with the fiber, eat lots of fruits like grapes, watermelon, and papaya, as well as vegetables which are high in fiber like okra and cabbage.

64.   If you have hemorrhoids, apply any brand of petroleum jelly directly on the affected area. This will help to ease the passing of any hard stools, and avoid causing further injury. Apply the jelly right before you feel the need to use the bathroom, and do this every time until your hemorrhoid is fully healed.

65.   To prevent hemorrhoids from getting worse, never ever use any type of dry toilet paper. If you do and you accidently scrape the hemorrhoid, this can cause you to bleed and be very uncomfortable. They sell wet wipes that are flushable, which would be a great alternative to standard paper.

66.   Regular daily exercise may help in the prevention and treatment of hemorrhoids. In our fast-paced world it can be hard to find time to fit exercise into our day but even a little can help. Try using the stairs instead of the elevator at work. Don't do any exercise that would cause straining, like lifting weights.

67.   If you are having issues with hemorrhoids, add a touch of lemon to the water that you drink. Lemon is filled with many soothing properties, and this can lower any irritation that you feel from hemorrhoids. Consume lemon water on a regular basis to help control your hemorrhoids.

68.   If you have a very firm chair at work, bring a cushion to sit on during the day. This cushion can reduce the amount of friction that you have on your skin, which can limit the sores that you acquire. Find a soft gel cushion to sit on while at work.

69.   If you have hemorrhoids, make sure that you do not scratch the affected area, regardless of how much it itches. Scratching can lead to extra irritation and redness, which can increase the longevity of your condition. Resisting the temptation of scratching will go a long way in improving your condition. Use a cream to lessen the itching. Wipe the area with wetwipes after a bowel movement. This also prevents irritation.

70.   If you are overweight, this can definitely lead to the development of hemorrhoids. When you have extra weight on your body, there is more pressure in your abdominal and waist area, as well as a high amount of pressure in the veins that are located in

the anus. Try to make sure that you are at a healthy weight for your size.

71.   To get rid of any swelling or pain try sitting in some hot warm water. Sitting in a tub with six to twelve inches of water, at lukewarm temperature, will increase blood flow and help reduce discomfort from hemorrhoids. Lift your knees into an upright position. Stay in the water at the very minimum until the water begins to lose temperature.

72.   Warm water can ease the suffering and pain from hemorrhoids. You can soak the area directly or take a soothing bath. Avoid using hot water as it can have a reverse effect than was intended. If you don't want to use warm water, a cold compress can also be used to provide relief.

73.   Hemorrhoid cushions can be really expensive, a great alternative to use is a soft pillow. A pillow has more give to it than the air inside of the rubber casing for a cusion. The air in the pillow can escape and will allow the pillow to conform to your bottom, whereas the rubber air-filled cushion will not conform quite as well.

74.   Don't expect laxatives or stool softeners to fix a hemorrhoid. Laxatives are not a long-term solution to the constipation issue that brought about the

hemorrhoid in the first place. Also, while a laxative may make the passing of stool easier, it doesn't actually fix the hemorrhoid. It simply reduces the symptoms.

75.   Witch hazel is one of the best over-the-counter medications to use when combating hemorrhoids. You can purchase this tonic at most any pharmacy store in your local area. The astringency of the witch hazel will reduce the bleeding and the swelling when it is applied.

76.   The first time you spot blood in your stool, you should never assume that this is from a hemorrhoid. Be sure that you visit a doctor to find out what's behind the blood in your stool. If it's bright red, then it's probably not internal bleeding, but you should never attempt to self-diagnose.

77.   Stay away from spicy and hot foods because they can inflame your hemorrhoids. Just making a few small changes in your diet can help you treat your current difficulties and help you prevent further complications. It is also important to limit the amount of coffee and beer that you drink.

78.   A great tip for your painful hemorrhoids is to stay away from lifting heavy items as much as you can. This is beneficial advice because you actually

end up using the same types of muscles that you would use when straining on the toilet and this can lead to increased pain.

79.   A great tip for your painful hemorrhoids is that you want to mix up your standing and sitting positions as much as possible throughout the day. This is good because you will even out the stress put on your hemorrhoid that occurs both when on your feet and sitting down.

80.   Add more fiber in your diet if you have hemorrhoids. Heavy straining during a bowel movement tends to cause hemorrhoids to develop. If you increase your fiber intake, you will avoid constipation and hard stools, both of which contribute to hemorrhoid problems. This can help prevent painful hemorrhoids.

81.   A great tip for your painful hemorrhoids is to try icing them. This is a great economical way to try to relieve the pain and itching of a hemorrhoid. Make sure you do not make direct contact with the ice and also either discard or thoroughly clean the applicator between sessions.

82.   A great tip for your painful hemorrhoids is to avoid any kind of strenuous exercise when you have them. You want to make sure that you rest as much

as possible and do not risk the possibility of further injuring yourself. Do not admit to others why you are taking a break, but give the workouts a rest for a few days.

83.   Apple cider vinegar is a safe and effective way to treat hemorrhoids. Soak a cotton ball with apple cider vinegar and apply to the area, leaving it on for several minutes. Do this a few times a day. You can also add apple cider vinegar to a warm sitz bath and soak for 20 minutes.

84.   Avoid hemorrhoids by eating a high-fiber diet. Fiber, especially soluble fiber, can help keep things moving without irritating your gastrointestinal tract. Examples of foods that are high in fiber, include cabbage, watermelon, and grapes. Increase your fiber intake slowly, to avoid shocking your system and backing things up even worse.

85.   To cure your hemorrhoids, try using yarrow tea. You can purchase yarrow tea from your local health food stores. To apply the yarrow tea, you should make the tea and let it brew for a half an hour to ensure its strength. Once the tea is finished brewing, absorb the yarrow tea with a cotton ball and apply to the hemorrhoids.

86.   Hemorrhoids can be very painful but cayenne is a natural remedy that can help. Cayenne is an incredible healing herb, stimulating the circulatory system and purifying the blood. Mix cayenne with coconut oil to make a paste and apply to the affected area. Drinking a cup of warm water with one-quarter to one-half teaspoon of cayenne will speed the healing process.

87.   A good option to treating a severe hemorrhoid problem is by using the herb horse chestnut. This herb was used in the past as a natural remedy to relieve swelling and inflammation. It can be taken as tea or in capsule form. It can also be applied externally as a compress. Before taking any supplement, be sure that you talk with your pharmacist or doctor.

88.   Do not spend too much time on the toilet waiting for a bowel movement to happen. It will only happen when your body is ready to make it happen. Sitting on the toilet reading a book for an hour is not going to help at all. Only try to go when you have the strong urge to go.

89.   You want to make sure you get yourself checked out by a physician, just so you know exactly what you're dealing with. There are much more serious causes of bloody stools, such as cancer, which

should be ruled out. Ease your worries by having a physician diagnose the problem. If it happens to be hemorrhoids, your doctor will tell you the best way to treat it.

90.   Make sure that you keep your body hydrated. Water is an excellent way to help alleviate some of the troublesome aspects of hemorrhoids. Water can help with constipation, one of the primary causes of hemorrhoids. Additionally, your body will be internally cleansed. Drink roughly eight glasses of water each and every day.

91.   Aloe Vera juice is a good drink to consume to help make the stools loose and easier to pass. If you don't like the way it tastes, try adding in a little apple juice. Follow the instructions on the label. Only consume the amount that is recommended. Just beware that excessive amounts of Aloe Vera juice could lead to stomach discomfort.

92.   It is ok to use a cream, but minimize the frequency. Many creams numb the pain caused by hemorrhoids, but they often won't alleviate swelling or irritation. Read the labels on any cream or ointment you choose to use, and seek your physicians advice if you feel you will exceed the package recommendations. If they are overused, they may cause more discomfort.

93.	If you are experiencing pain and inflammation from your hemorrhoids, try to soak in a warm tub. Fill your tub with enough warm water to cover the area and lay back with your knees raised. The warm water will increase the blood flow to the anus and reduce the swelling. Do this a few times a day to help reduce the swelling.

94.	The most effective way to prevent hemorrhoids is to make sure your stool is not hard. Having to push out hard stools will irritate your anus, and ultimately, cause hemorrhoids. Try to eat foods that contain a lot of fiber, such as vegetables, and purchase a stool softener if needed.

95.	Warm water can ease the suffering and pain from hemorrhoids. You can soak the area directly or take a soothing bath. Avoid using hot water as it can have a reverse effect than was intended. If you don't want to use warm water, a cold compress can also be used to provide relief.

96.	Exercise is a great way in which you can work to soften your stools. If you feel like you have to strain to use the bathroom, this is going to be bad for your hemorrhoid. You're in no danger of having an accident if you can't get it out anyway, so go ahead and take a long walk or jog.

97.   There are products sold over the counter called hemorrhoid pads. These can be effective against flareups. Both men and women can safely use these pads. They're similar to the sanitary pads women wear when they are having their periods.

98.   An important part of managing your hemorrhoids is to make sure that your diet is high in fiber. Because it can often be difficult for Americans to get adequate amounts of fiber in their diet, consider taking a fiber supplement, and drink plenty of water with your supplement to avoid constipation.

99.   Take note of your salt intake when struggling with hemorrhoids. Consuming lots of salt can cause the body and hemorrhoids to swell. If your food seems too bland without using salt there are many spices and herbs that will add new and exciting flavors to your foods without the effects of added salt.

100.   When dealing with hemorrhoids, you should not sit or stand for too long. You should try to alternate between sitting and standing throughout the day. When you sit or stand for long periods of time, you are increasing the pressure on your hemorrhoids. This can cause the hemorrhoids to become worse.

101.   If you are prone to hemorrhoids and you have a job that requires a lot of sitting, then you need to get up and move a few minutes each hour. Exercise is very important in the prevention and treatment of hemorrhoids. Also, you will want to refrain from heavy lifting and anal intercourse to avoid the risk of developing hemorrhoids.

102.   One way to relieve your hemorrhoids is to apply ice to your hemorrhoid to help relieve pain. This is a cost effective method of relieving pain that only takes a little bit of money. Keep your life comfortable when you control your hemorrhoids by applying ice to the affected area.

103.   It is very important to get the proper nutrients in your body if you are trying to reduce the symptoms of hemorrhoids. When you wake up in the morning eat an orange or an apple. These fruits will give you the vitamins that you need to improve blood circulation for your hemorrhoids.

104.   If you have hemorrhoids and find that your problem hasn't taken care of itself after a couple of weeks or the problem seems to be getting worse quickly than you should go to a professional immediately. Probably you will have no major

problems but they will be able to tell you exactly what is going on.

105.   Eat fiber! One of the best solutions to treating hemorrhoids is by adding more fiber to your diet! Fiber will keep your stool soft and decrease bulk which will help reduce straining. Studies have shown that the increase of fiber in a diet will improve the discomfort of itching and pain associated with hemorrhoids.

106.   Take a fiber supplement. Fiber will help to soften your stool but if you do not enjoy eating fruits and vegetables, you will not get a recommended amount of fiber. When taking a fiber supplement, you should always make sure to keep up with your fluid intake or it may cause more problems.

107.   Lifting any type of heavy object is not good for your body, and can lead to hemorrhoids. The stress of lifting anything that is too heavy for you, even if you only do it once, is the same thing that happens to your body when you are pushing too hard when trying to go to the bathroom.

108.   A great way to ease your hemorrhoid problems is to lose weight. The excess weight around your abdomen and waist areas increase the pressure put

on the veins in and around the anus. If you lose this excess weight it will relieve the pressure in this area and help with your hemorrhoid problems.

109.   Apply a cream occasionally. While they don't actually provide any treatment, they do slightly numb the affected area. Check with your doctor if you feel the need to use them for longer than a week. Applying them too much can cause extra pain, particularly if applied more often than is allowed.

110.   Overweight individuals are at a bigger risk for hemorrhoids, so you should lose weight if you want to reduce your risk or reduce the swelling of a pre-existing hemorrhoid. A larger waist and abdominal area means that you are putting g a lot more weight on the veins in your rectum.

111.   If you suffer from chronic or repeated hemorrhoids, try losing some weight. Carrying extra weight, especially around the waist and hips, puts extra pressure on your abdominal cavity. This can then translate to increased pressure in the blood vessels in the anal area, resulting in exacerbation of your hemorrhoid issue.

112.   Try squatting when you go to the toilet rather than sitting upon the seat. It will make the

movement pass easier, plus it will stop painful flare-ups of hemorrhoids. Of course, it will take a while to get used to. But after you begin squatting, you will find that you're experiencing fewer flare-ups due to less swelling and irritation.

113.   Some everyday products work wonders for hemorrhoids, and using something as simple and affordable as apple cider vinegar can help you to heal hemorrhoids. The acid in the vinegar will help you in the digestion of your food, and this will ultimately create smaller, looser bowel movements that will not cause your veins to become irritated.

114.   Stay away from spicy and hot foods because they can inflame your hemorrhoids. Just making a few small changes in your diet can help you treat your current difficulties and help you prevent further complications. It is also important to limit the amount of coffee and beer that you drink.

115.   A great tip for your painful hemorrhoids is to cut back on how much sodium you consume. This is essential because salt dries out your body, and this is the worst thing you can do to yourself if you are already suffering from difficult and painful bowel movements. On a side note, salt is not good for your heart health either.

116.   One of the most common causes of hemorrhoid formation is chronic bouts of constipation. Preventing constipation and encouraging more regular bowel movements can go a long way in avoiding both internal and external hemorrhoids. Look for natural constipation remedies, such as aloe vera juice. Aloe vera can also be taken in gel or capsule form.

117.   To reduce the pain and swelling associated with hemorrhoids, you should soak in warm water. To do this, you need to fill a bathtub with six to 12 inches of warm water. After your tub is filled, sit in the water with your knees elevated. Doing this several times a day will increase the results. The warm water will improve the blood flow to the area.

118.   Your diet can have a significant impact on whether or not you are more prone to suffering from hemorrhoids. Certain foods and drinks can be especially irritating as they pass through the bowels. A diet that is filled with overly spicy foods or strong beverages like coffee, soda, and alcohol will put you at greater risk of forming hemorrhoids.

119.   There are two types of hemorrhoids that are common in humans and while they have many similarities there are also several key differences. The most common and easiest type of this is an

external hemorrhoid which is really not all that different from a varicose vein and can be treated very easily.

120.   If you have a hemorrhoid problem, you may want to consider applying petroleum jelly to your rectum before trying to make a bowel movement. This can help smoothen the passage of hard stools and will help to avoid damaging the hemorrhoids that you already have and avoid getting any more.

121.   If you get hemorrhoids it is important to get exercise and move around throughout your day. If you are sedentary, and constantly sitting, you are putting much unneeded pressure on the veins which can become hemorrhoids. If your work is sedentary, get up often and walk around. Keep your lifestyle active to help prevent hemorrhoids!

122.   Don't depend on medications. Stimulant laxative drugs such as Bisacodyl tablets are meant to be used on a short-term basis and will not cure constipation. They may help with one bowel movement, but you'll be more constipated later. Side effects may include upset stomach, diarrhea, stomach cramps, faintness and stomach & intestinal irritation.

123.   Use moist toilet tissue or non-alcohol wipes when cleaning yourself on the toilet. Dry paper

equates to rough paper no matter the softness of the tissue. The paper can cause bleeding from the hemorrhoids and should be avoided if possible. If you have access to a bidet you can use this as an alternative for paper.

124. See a doctor if your hemorrhoids are too painful or large. There are safe and simple surgical procedures, often done in your doctor's office or in an outpatient clinic. Treatments include a shot into the hemorrhoid to reduce swelling (sclerotherapy), a rubber band around it to cut off its blood supply, shrinking it with heat, freezing it with liquid nitrogen and minor surgery (hemorrhoidectomy).

125. Use moist towelettes instead of regular toilet paper. Some toilet paper brands can be tough and dry, which can increase itching and pain. By using a moist towelette, you can provide relief to the painful area. Avoid using paper towel on your rectal area, as they are usually rough and not intended for sensitive skin.

126. It might seem like a cheap trick you can use for practically any pain and that's because it is, but a simple ice pack will work wonders to help ease the pain associated with hemorrhoid flare-ups. You can use one of those cooler ice packs or simply put some ice in a plastic bag.

127.   Anything that puts increased pressure on the veins in your rectum is something you want to avoid with hemorrhoids. This even includes sitting or standing for too long. Yes, it doesn't sound like it would matter, but standing up can actually put a strain on the veins in your rectum.

128.   Constipation can contribute to the development of hemorrhoids or make them worse if you currently have them. Consume a diet rich in high-fiber foods or take a fiber supplement every day. Drink plenty of water along with the extra fiber as this will help your stool to become softer and easier to pass.

129.   Eat whole wheat bread to facilitate the digestive process. As an added benefit, whole wheat will also help to reduce general skin irritation. Replace white bread and pasta with wheat products and eat brown rice instead of white rice.

130.   Hemorrhoid relief is as close as the nearest bottle of witch hazel. Witch hazel provides instant relief from the pain and itching caused by hemorrhoids via its unique numbing quality. While witch hazel is not necessarily a magic cure for hemorrhoids, it does greatly relieve those tissues and gives them a chance to heal.

131.   If you are suffering from hemorrhoids then you may want to consider purchasing some witch hazel. You can apply the witch hazel to them topically. Witch hazel has been shown to effectively reduce the size if hemorrhoids which in consequence lessens the itching and pain that you will suffer because of them.

132.   If you find that you are in constant pain from hemorrhoids and you are overweight, you may want to consider starting a serious diet and fitness routine. If you can lose some weight, you will eliminate some of the pressure that the extra weight is putting on the veins that are in the anus, which causes the hemorrhoids.

133.   It is important for you to have a bowel movement when you feel the urge, if you put it off this can lead to constipation as well as encourage the development of hemorrhoids. Put yourself first, and take time for yourself when you feel the urge to defecate. By doing this, you can possibly avoid getting painful hemorrhoids.

134.   You should definitely avoid, spicy or hot foods, and caffeine is also on the list of things to avoid. This kind of foods can irritate your intestine and worsen your hemorrhoids. In fact, eating spicy

foods can inflame hemorrhoids to a point of painful burning, so steer clear of them if you don't want to spend all your time in the bathroom.

135.   To ease some of the pain and discomfort of hemorrhoids, lay in a warm bath that is filled with about six to twelve inches of water. After you have soaked for about five minuets, sit in the tub with your knees raised. This will reduce any swelling, and you should repeat this several times a day.

136.   To alleviate the swelling and pain, try sitting in a warm tub of water. Fill the tub with approximately six inches or more of water at a medium warm temperature. This will greatly reduce the discomfort of hemorrhoidal flareups. Keep your knees elevated. Don't be afraid to stay in the tub until the water cools.

137.   A great way to ease your hemorrhoid problems is to lose weight. The excess weight around your abdomen and waist areas increase the pressure put on the veins in and around the anus. If you lose this excess weight it will relieve the pressure in this area and help with your hemorrhoid problems.

138.   Hemorrhoids are a common and irritating complication of pregnancy. It's important to avoid any natural or over-the-counter remedies until you

consult with your doctor to see what is safe for you and your baby. Try sleeping on your left side to reduce pressure on certain veins that can make hemorrhoids swell.

139. Anything that puts increased pressure on the veins in your rectum is something you want to avoid with hemorrhoids. This even includes sitting or standing for too long. Yes, it doesn't sound like it would matter, but standing up can actually put a strain on the veins in your rectum.

140. If you are suffering from an extremely painful hemorrhoid, try soaking in a warm bath. Doctors recommend sitting in about six to twelve inches of water with your knees raised. Doing this can improve circulating in the hemorrhoid, which will reduce the swelling and also the pain. You can also try a sitz bath, which can be purchased at any medical supply store.

141. After getting out of the bath or shower, try to avoid drying your rectum with a towel if you hope to avoid any hemorrhoid pain associated with flare-ups. Instead, opt for air-drying the area. This may take a little while longer, but you will most definitely appreciate the results here.

142.   Change your diet to include less salt. If you eat foods that are high in salt, it can make many different parts of your body swell, including your hemorrhoids. Reducing your salt intake can improve and prevent hemorrhoids, as well as lower your blood pressure. Not only will it be easier to use the restroom, but you will feel healthier overall.

143.   A great tip for your painful hemorrhoids is to be sure that you drink plenty of water each day. This will aid in your ability to easily pass bowel movements. If you are hydrated, everything in your body will flow much more efficiently and you will feel much better about yourself.

144.   If you find yourself having re-occurring hemorrhoids, you should make sure that you are drinking at least 8 glasses of water a day. Constipation can be caused by not getting enough fluids, and it is the most likely cause of the hemorrhoids. Drinking enough water in addition to getting a variety of fiber, may be enough to prevent them from coming back in the future.

145.   Doctors agree that including more fiber in your diet goes a long way in preventing hemorrhoids. You should eat whole grain foods, pasta, oatmeal and a lot of leafy green vegetables. Fiber will ease

your bowel movements and remove the pressure put on your hemorrhoids.

146.   A simple remedy you can use at home is applying ice, then heat. This has the effect of shrinking the hemorrhoid. Our advice is to apply the ice pack first for a quarter of an hour, then use warmth for about twenty minutes.

147.   One way to help relieve your hemorrhoid pain is to take a warm bath. The hot water will help relieve the itching sensation and the pain. Additionally, when you take a bath, you are eliminating the bacteria that can cause your hemorrhoids to worsen, keeping your body healthy and happy.

148.   Another way that you can relieve the pain caused from your hemorrhoid is to go on a diet with lots of fruits and vegetables. These sorts of diets are high in fiber, which helps to keep your bowel movements soft. This will relieve the irritation caused by your daily defecation.

149.   Wheat bread is wonderful for your digestion, and can also improve hemorrhoids. It also reduces the redness and irritation of your skin. Replace white bread and pasta with wheat products and eat brown rice instead of white rice.

150.   If you have hemorrhoids and find that your problem hasn't taken care of itself after a couple of weeks or the problem seems to be getting worse quickly than you should go to a professional immediately. Probably you will have no major problems but they will be able to tell you exactly what is going on.

151.   If you have a very firm chair at work, bring a cushion to sit on during the day. This cushion can reduce the amount of friction that you have on your skin, which can limit the sores that you acquire. Find a soft gel cushion to sit on while at work.

152.   Do not spend too much time on the toilet waiting for a bowel movement to happen. It will only happen when your body is ready to make it happen. Sitting on the toilet reading a book for an hour is not going to help at all. Only try to go when you have the strong urge to go.

153.   If constipation is a big problem, you are going to have more hemorrhoids. Consider taking a good fiber supplement. This supplement will soften your stool and make it easier for you to pass bowel movements. This is great for the people that do not like to eat fruits and vegetables on a regular basis.

154.   To promote softer stools, you should drink as much water as possible and increase your intake of fiber. If your stool has been softened, there will be less strain during movements so that can help to stop hemorrhoids occurring. You can increase your consumption of specific fruits, such as papaya or watermelon, to help naturally soften your stool. Vegetables with high fiber content, like cabbage, also help keep the stools soft. Adequate amounts of water every day helps these foods be more effective.

155.   If you have hemorrhoids, make sure that you do not scratch the affected area, regardless of how much it itches. Scratching can lead to extra irritation and redness, which can increase the longevity of your condition. Resisting the temptation of scratching will go a long way in improving your condition. Use a cream to lessen the itching. Wipe the area with wetwipes after a bowel movement. This also prevents irritation.

156.   You need to limit the amount of salt in your diet in order to reduce or prevent hemorrhoids. Too much salt will lead to fluid retention, which in turn will cause your body to swell, which includes the blood vessels that actually cause hemorrhoids. By making some changes in your diet, decreasing salt and increasing fluid intake, you may be able to prevent getting hemorrhoids.

157.   Reducing your salt intake is key to helping with your hemorrhoid problems. Not only is salt bad for your blood pressure, but salt increases swelling in the body. This swelling will happen throughout the entire body including the hemorrhoid area. The hemorrhoids swelling is what causes a majority of pain and suffering.

158.   Lay on your side to alleviate pressure. Sitting upright or laying on your back may inadvertently cause more pressure to the rectal area, so relieve that pressure by laying and sleeping on your side. This is especially true for hemorrhoids caused by pregnancy, and the expanding uterus is pulled down toward the rectal area, causing more pressure.

159.   If you have been having chronic hemorrhoid pain and it does not seem to ever get better, see your doctor. There are surgical procedures that are very safe and simple that can help with hemorrhoids.

160.   It is a good idea to go to your doctor and have the area checked out. The blood you see on your toilet paper or in your stool might be from a more serious condition.

161. Olive oil is a terrific home remedy for hemorrhoids. Olive oil, as strange as it may seem, is known for its ability to reduce swelling and relieve itching caused by hemorrhoids. However, only use olive oil to treat external hemorrhoids. Avoid using the oil to treat internal hemorrhoids.

162. If you are prone to getting hemorrhoids, then you want to be sure that you are drinking enough water. Your stools will be softer and easier to pass when you are properly hydrated. Avoid both alcohol and caffeine to avoid dehydration.

163. Although or perhaps especially because this problem can be a bit uncomfortable for many people to talk about it is essential that you know what is going on and feel comfortable talking to a medical professional. Remember that they have seen much stranger problems many times throughout their life and career.

164. Avoid foods that are very high in sugar to reduce the symptoms of hemorrhoids. Sugars can expedite the formation of hemorrhoids and can make you feel very uncomfortable during the day. Find alternatives to foods that have high carbohydrates and sugars if you want to reduce irritation and skin redness.

165.   One of the best things that you can put on your skin to improve your condition, is vitamin E oil. Vitamin E helps to soothe and smooth out the surface of your skin, which can help your hemorrhoids. If you prefer, you can take vitamin E in a capsule, as well.

166.   Experiment with natural home remedies before shelling out cash for expensive treatments and medications. If you have just had a bowel movement, try relaxing in a lukewarm sitz bath for around 15 minutes. Hemorrhoids are often incredibly itchy, but do your best to avoid scratching them, as this can only worsen the problem overall. Instead, use witch hazel to dampen some pads and apply them on the hemorrhoids to get relief. Stay hydrated by drinking plenty of water, and eat foods that are high in fiber. This will help eliminate strain from your bowel movements.

167.   Hemorrhoid relief is as close as the nearest bottle of witch hazel. Witch hazel provides instant relief from the pain and itching caused by hemorrhoids via its unique numbing quality. While witch hazel is not necessarily a magic cure for hemorrhoids, it does greatly relieve those tissues and gives them a chance to heal.

168.   If you suffer from hemorrhoids, keep protein in your diet at a minimum. Protein tends to bind stool and hard stools lead to straining when going to the bathroom. That straining not only helps cause hemorrhoids, but also leads to much pain when using the toilet. Keep your stools soft by eating plenty of fruits, vegetables and fiber.

169.   If you are suffering from hemorrhoids then you may want to consider purchasing some witch hazel. You can apply the witch hazel to them topically. Witch hazel has been shown to effectively reduce the size if hemorrhoids which in consequence lessens the itching and pain that you will suffer because of them.

170.   Cut back on your salt intake. Salt can make your body swell including your hemorrhoids. Reducing your salt intake may be difficult at first but will be well worth it in the end.

171.   If you think you might be constipated, try taking a walk prior to going to the restroom. This can prepare your body for your next bowel movement. This will help you not to have to strain as you have a movement, reducing your risk of hemorrhoids or the condition getting worse. Try a brisk 15 minute walk.

172.   Many people like to read while sitting on the toilet. This is a perfect way to get hemorrhoids. You can be sitting much longer than you need to be, and pushing a little harder without even realizing it. If you are sitting longer than 5 minutes without anything happening, you have been sitting too long.

173.   Always clean your anal area carefully and meticulously. With hemorrhoids present, the likelihood of infection can increase. Bacteria can cause abscesses through infected tissue. Wash after bowel movements and always in the shower. Clean the area thoroughly with soap and make sure to rinse any soap residue away to avoid discomfort.

174.   Caffeine, along with spicy foods, should be avoided when you have hemorrhoids. These types of foods can cause intestinal irritation, which in turn can make hemorrhoids worse. Foods that are very spicy could affect hemorrhoids so badly that they have burning sensation, even when you are out of the restroom. So avoiding them can certainly improve your well-being.

175.   If you are suffering through a bout of hemorrhoids, you should think about getting a donut cushion for your comfort. This cushion is designed specifically to provide maximum comfort

for your bottom. Just sitting on that will make you more relaxed and in less pain.

176.   Doctors suggest that using a little petroleum jelly can help ease the pain of hemorrhoids. Before you defecate, smear a little petroleum jelly around the anus. This should help the passage of the stools. If it is a particularly hard stool, a little petroleum jelly can help avoid any injuries to the hemorrhoids.

177.   The most effective way to prevent hemorrhoids is to make sure your stool is not hard. Having to push out hard stools will irritate your anus, and ultimately, cause hemorrhoids. Try to eat foods that contain a lot of fiber, such as vegetables, and purchase a stool softener if needed.

178.   Applying ointment directly to a hemorrhoid is a good way to help shrink the size of it. A hemorrhoid is a swollen, possibly ruptured vein, so a medicine like Neosporin can help to heal the sore partially. It will not completely remove the hemorrhoid, but it will help in reducing the size.

179.   Apple cider vinegar is a safe and effective way to treat hemorrhoids. Soak a cotton ball with apple cider vinegar and apply to the area, leaving it on for several minutes. Do this a few times a day. You can

also add apple cider vinegar to a warm sitz bath and soak for 20 minutes.

180.   When trying to cure hemorrhoids, be sure to take note of which medicines you are taking. Most laxatives will not help with hemorrhoids. They are designed to help with one bowel movement. Laxatives may leave you more constipated after that first bowel movement. Many laxatives are not designed for helping with hemorrhoids.

181.   When you need to have a bowel movement, try applying petroleum jelly around your anus before using the bathroom. Using petroleum jelly around the anus will help the passage of hard stools go more smoothly. This technique can help you avoid injuring your hemorrhoids. It can be very painful to injure your hemorrhoids and this should help you prevent that.

182.   Are you looking for immediate relief of your hemorrhoids without purchasing over-the-counter medication? If you have an aloe vera plant in your home or garden, this plant offer immediate relief for the pain and swelling associated with hemorrhoids. Simply break a leaf from the plant and rub the juice from the leaf on the affected area. It will reduce the inflammation and have a soothing effect on your hemorrhoids.

183.   You may think that you are alone in this problem and that it is something to be embarrassed about, but it actually occurs in almost half of all adults by the time they reach middle age. Their are many products available which can help greatly with this issue available over the counter because it is so common.

184.   Cut back on your salt intake. Salt can make your body swell including your hemorrhoids. Reducing your salt intake may be difficult at first but will be well worth it in the end.

185.   You need to limit the amount of salt in your diet in order to reduce or prevent hemorrhoids. Too much salt will lead to fluid retention, which in turn will cause your body to swell, which includes the blood vessels that actually cause hemorrhoids. By making some changes in your diet, decreasing salt and increasing fluid intake, you may be able to prevent getting hemorrhoids.

186.   Hemorrhoids can come around during pregnancy because of all the extra weight and stress that your body is carrying around. It is best to lay on your left side if you are going through this for 20 minutes every five hours so that the blood vessels

of your hemorrhoids can get some relief from the pressure of your uterus.

187.   Use petroleum jelly liberally. Applying petroleum jelly around your anus before you use the restroom can alleviate any pain you may experience from the passage of hard stools. It lubricates and soothes, saving you from experiencing pain and discomfort both during and after your restroom break by preventing inflammation of the hemorrhoids.

188.   Never scratch. While hemorrhoids are known for being terribly itchy, scratching at it is the last thing you want to do. You will not only cause more irritation and inflammation, but you may cause tears that allow bacteria to get in. You may also end up with fecal material under your fingernails.

189.   Make sure to keep your anal area clean in order to prevent hemorrhoids. One of the causes of hemorrhoids is lack of hygiene. Be sure to wipe well after a bowel movement. Also, when you are in the shower be sure to clean your anal area, but do not rub too hard.

190.   Eating too much salt can cause you to retain a lot of water and thus increase your odds of swelling, including that hemorrhoid! Your veins can swell

with too much salt and that pain and discomfort will return. Reduce your salt to reduce the size and pain associated with hemorrhoids.

191.   Avoid spicy foods such as chilies and similar spices. These spices are harsh and irritating on the sensitive lining of your bowels, and are persistent enough to cause an issue at the point of the hemorrhoid. If you do eat spicy foods, combine them with a cooling dairy product, such as sour cream, to reduce the problem.

192.   When it comes to the many tips you'll read in your lifetime, you'll find that a lot of them have to do with water in some form or another, and it's no different with this hemorrhoid tip. If you want to help out your hemorrhoid, drink a lot of water to keep your digestive tract lubricated and your stools moving along nicely.

193.   You can reduce swelling and pain from hemorrhoids by eating grape seed oil. That way, you can naturally eradicate vein infections and halt the bleeding of your hemorrhoids.

194.   Make sure you use a lenient exercise program. Weight lifting and consistent sweating can cause your hemorrhoid pain and swelling to worsen, so try to stick with less strenuous exercises, such as

walking, swimming, or yoga. Yoga is encouraged, as light stretching can be greatly beneficial to your intestinal muscles and overall health.

195.   A great tip for your painful hemorrhoids is to consider seeing a doctor if you notice any extreme increase in pain. This is important because it could be a symptom of something worse that might require surgery. Your doctor is a professional and it will be less embarrassing than you imagine.

196.   If you prefer more natural ingredients for treating your ailments, consider purchasing a salve, ointment, or cream that contains horse chestnut. This botanical product, which is very popular in European countries, can be applied directly to external hemorrhoids. Within minutes, the topical solution will shrink the size of the hemorrhoid and offer relief from stinging sensations.

197.   Hemorrhoid relief is as close as the nearest bottle of witch hazel. Witch hazel provides instant relief from the pain and itching caused by hemorrhoids via its unique numbing quality. While witch hazel is not necessarily a magic cure for hemorrhoids, it does greatly relieve those tissues and gives them a chance to heal.

198.   If you are suffering from hemorrhoids then you may want to consider purchasing some witch hazel. You can apply the witch hazel to them topically. Witch hazel has been shown to effectively reduce the size if hemorrhoids which in consequence lessens the itching and pain that you will suffer because of them.

199.   If you get hemorrhoids it is important to get exercise and move around throughout your day. If you are sedentary, and constantly sitting, you are putting much unneeded pressure on the veins which can become hemorrhoids. If your work is sedentary, get up often and walk around. Keep your lifestyle active to help prevent hemorrhoids!

200.   Try using an ice pack to reduce swelling and alleviate pain from a hemorrhoid flareup. Some people also find applying over the counter creams or witch hazel to the affected area helpful in reducing swelling. To prevent further hemorrhoid irritation use a donut pillow when sitting or avoid sitting altogether.

201.   Lose a little weight. Hemorrhoids are most common in people who are overweight, so dropping a few pounds can make all the difference. Incorporating ten to fifteen minutes of exercise into

your daily routine is an easy way to both lose weight and keep any painful hemorrhoid issues at bay.

202. If you have hemorrhoids, apply any brand of petroleum jelly directly on the affected area. This will help to ease the passing of any hard stools, and avoid causing further injury. Apply the jelly right before you feel the need to use the bathroom, and do this every time until your hemorrhoid is fully healed.

203. Never lift heavy items. Lifting something heavy actually puts the same pressure on your rectum as straining to defecate. If you already have hemorrhoids, you may be irritating them by lifting and carrying heavy objects, so always make sure you are using correct lifting methods, or pairing up when you know something may be too heavy.

204. In order to reduce the pain and suffering of your hemorrhoid problem, you need to stop eating spicy foods. The capsaicin oil in hot peppers does not digest fully after traveling through your body. So what is hot going in, is just as hot coming out, and oftentimes worse because it will cover your hemorrhoids on exiting your body.

205. You should consult a medical professional if you experience prolonged or excessive bleeding from

hemorrhoids. In rare cases excessive blood loss from hemorrhoids has caused anemia and alternative treatments like surgery or rubber band ligation may be required to treat hemorrhoids. It is also possible that the bleeding indicates a more serious condition that needs immediate medical attention.

206.   Keep it as clean as possible. If your hemorrhoid breaks open and bleeds, and then becomes dirty, it could get infected. You could eventually get an abscess in the are, requiring medical attention or surgery. Use a damp, clean cloth to gently clean the area when you bathe, so as not to inflame it.

207.   If you are suffering from an extremely painful hemorrhoid, try soaking in a warm bath. Doctors recommend sitting in about six to twelve inches of water with your knees raised. Doing this can improve circulating in the hemorrhoid, which will reduce the swelling and also the pain. You can also try a sitz bath, which can be purchased at any medical supply store.

208.   After getting out of the bath or shower, try to avoid drying your rectum with a towel if you hope to avoid any hemorrhoid pain associated with flare-ups. Instead, opt for air-drying the area. This may

take a little while longer, but you will most definitely appreciate the results here.

209.   A great tip for your painful hemorrhoids is that you should lie on our side as often as possible if you are suffering while pregnant. This is a great tip because it will relieve a lot of the pressure from your anal area that is being caused by an enlarged uterus.

210.   A great tip for your painful hemorrhoids is to consider seeing a doctor if you notice any extreme increase in pain. This is important because it could be a symptom of something worse that might require surgery. Your doctor is a professional and it will be less embarrassing than you imagine.

211.   A great tip for your painful hemorrhoids is to use apple cider vinegar directly on the hemorrhoid itself. This is a good natural way to try to fix this awful condition you are experiencing. Use a cotton swab and apply directly to the area and as often as needed within reason.

212.   Witch hazel is an excellent way to treat the discomfort that goes along with hemorrhoids. Astringent witch hazel contracts hemorrhoid tissue, which bring a sigh of relief to sufferers. Use cotton balls to apply witch hazel, and allow it to sit on the

affected area for somewhere between 5 and 10 minutes, or simply pour some into your sitz bath.

213.   Try to limit the amount of sitting that you do during the course of the day. Remaining stagnant in your seat can lead to a lot of irritation and can strain your affected area of skin. If you are at work, limit the sitting that you do to improve your condition.

214.   Although or perhaps especially because this problem can be a bit uncomfortable for many people to talk about it is essential that you know what is going on and feel comfortable talking to a medical professional. Remember that they have seen much stranger problems many times throughout their life and career.

215.   There are several uncomfortable symptoms that can come about as a result of this issue and it is important that you face each of them head on. The most common and perhaps first sign of developing hemorrhoids is bleeding during bowel movements. This is always a sign that something is not working properly.

216.   After you take a shower, make sure that the area of your hemorrhoids is completely dry. Putting clothes on a wet body can lead to excess irritation during the course of the day, which can be very

painful. Prevent this by using a soft towel that captures all moisture on your body after washing.

217.   Hot and spicy foods are going to react badly with your hemorrhoids. The spices that are in foods like chili are going to irritate the hemorrhoids and cause you a great deal of pain. If you are suffering from a break out of hemorrhoids, eliminate these spicy foods from your diet and you should notice a reduction in pain.

218.   Lifting any type of heavy object is not good for your body, and can lead to hemorrhoids. The stress of lifting anything that is too heavy for you, even if you only do it once, is the same thing that happens to your body when you are pushing too hard when trying to go to the bathroom.

219.   Standing for long periods of time without moving can cause hemorrhoids to form. The same problem can occur if you are sitting for hours on end and not getting up for a break. Try alternating between sitting and standing if you are not able to get up and walk around during the day.

220.   Hemorrhoids have been known to be incredibly itchy and uncomfortable when healing. No matter how miserable it is, you must never scratch them. If you scratch, you can lead to scraping and bleeding.

The worst possibility is that you can cause the wound to fully open and become infected and even more uncomfortable and painful.

221.   Hemorrhoids can come around during pregnancy because of all the extra weight and stress that your body is carrying around. It is best to lay on your left side if you are going through this for 20 minutes every five hours so that the blood vessels of your hemorrhoids can get some relief from the pressure of your uterus.

222.   If you are experiencing pain and inflammation from your hemorrhoids, try to soak in a warm tub. Fill your tub with enough warm water to cover the area and lay back with your knees raised. The warm water will increase the blood flow to the anus and reduce the swelling. Do this a few times a day to help reduce the swelling.

223.   Be sure to stay away from alcohol if you want to avoid developing hemorrhoids. Too much alcohol, even wine, can cause your to become dehydrated. Dehydration is one of the many causes of hemorrhoids. Also, alcohol causes constipation, which causes hemorrhoids because you have to push your stools out too hard.

224.   It is extremely important to drink lots of water if you have hemorrhoids. Most people don't drink enough. But water keeps you hydrated and helps to create a soft stool that is easy to pass. Also keep in mind that caffeine and alcohol deplete the body of water and can contribute to constipation.

225.   A natural remedy you can use in order to prevent hemorrhoids is red sage. This is a Chinese herb that helps with blood circulation. Improper blood flow is one of the causes of hemorrhoids. In addition to red sage, you can use Vitamin E. This helps to protect against rectal damage.

226.   Hot cayenne pepper is a great tool for preventing hemorrhoid. Many times, hemorrhoids form because the body is not getting enough circulation. Hot cayenne pepper helps circulate blood throughout your whole body, even to the anal area. Horse chestnut and butcher's broom are natural ingredients that have the same purpose.

227.   If your constipation has given you hemorrhoids, you'll need to address this cause before you see any relief. Straining to have a bowel movement can often cause hemorrhoids, so switching to a high-fiber diet may make things move through your system more easily. Apple cider vinegar is an effective natural laxative that can help.

228.   Hemorrhoid cushions can be really expensive, a great alternative to use is a soft pillow. A pillow has more give to it than the air inside of the rubber casing for a cusion. The air in the pillow can escape and will allow the pillow to conform to your bottom, whereas the rubber air-filled cushion will not conform quite as well.

229.   If you have an aloe vera plant, you can break off a piece and use the gel as a soothing salve or compress that can be applied to painful and swollen external hemorrhoids. Break the stem, then gently squeeze it repeatedly to extract the maximal amount of gel. The gel can then be applied directly to the hemorrhoid.

230.   One common cause of recurrent hemorrhoids is a failure to consume enough water. Your stools will be softer if you are hydrated. Try to limit your caffeine and alcohol intake, too.

231.   You may think that you are alone in this problem and that it is something to be embarrassed about, but it actually occurs in almost half of all adults by the time they reach middle age. Their are many products available which can help greatly with this issue available over the counter because it is so common.

232.   The first line of defense against this
uncomfortable problem is actually a very simple
over the counter cream which can be purchased at
all drug stores and most super markets. This will
help with the inflammation and pain and the actual
hemorrhoid will take care of itself in up to two
weeks.

233.   Avoid foods that are very high in sugar to
reduce the symptoms of hemorrhoids. Sugars can
expedite the formation of hemorrhoids and can
make you feel very uncomfortable during the day.
Find alternatives to foods that have high
carbohydrates and sugars if you want to reduce
irritation and skin redness.

234.   Smoking is one of the worst things that you can
do if you have hemorrhoids because it will hurt the
quality of your immune system. This will directly
impact your hemorrhoids, causing more irritation
and redness on your skin. Reduce or quit smoking
entirely to improve your condition and well-being.

235.   If you have hemorrhoids, add mint to the water
that you drink. Mint has very soothing
characteristics and can calm you down when you
are stressed. This can improve your condition and
help you get your hemorrhoids under control.

Drink mint water to help you feel better during the day.

236.   Although it may not be commonly known, lifting heavy objects can lead to hemorrhoids. The strain of lifting heavy objects is similar to the strain required to force feces out of the body. If you regularly lift heavy objects and have recurring hemorrhoids, find ways to avoid doing this lifting.

237.   Hot and spicy foods are going to react badly with your hemorrhoids. The spices that are in foods like chili are going to irritate the hemorrhoids and cause you a great deal of pain. If you are suffering from a break out of hemorrhoids, eliminate these spicy foods from your diet and you should notice a reduction in pain.

238.   You should consult a medical professional if you experience prolonged or excessive bleeding from hemorrhoids. In rare cases excessive blood loss from hemorrhoids has caused anemia and alternative treatments like surgery or rubber band ligation may be required to treat hemorrhoids. It is also possible that the bleeding indicates a more serious condition that needs immediate medical attention.

239.   If hemorrhoids come out, try to gently push them back in. Wash your hands thoroughly before attempting this to avoid introducing foreign bacteria that could cause infection and inflammation. After this happens, you should schedule an appointment with your doctor immediately, but if they are not too swollen, you can prevent any further damage.

240.   Applying ointment directly to a hemorrhoid is a good way to help shrink the size of it. A hemorrhoid is a swollen, possibly ruptured vein, so a medicine like Neosporin can help to heal the sore partially. It will not completely remove the hemorrhoid, but it will help in reducing the size.

241.   As far as products go, there are plenty of treatments that you can choose from when it comes to your hemorrhoids and one of the best is a numbing topical spray that you can purchase. This spray is easy to apply and works to numb the pain. It won't really help it to heal, but it will numb the pain.

242.   If you're attempting to clean your rectal area in the bath or shower to manage your hemorrhoid, make sure you're using a gentle cleaning product and not some perfumed soap that may cause a lot of drying, itching and burning. Cleaning should

never make the hemorrhoid worse, so watch what you're cleaning with.

243.   Some people think that a hemorrhoid pillow can offer relief from their suffering, but in fact, sitting on a donut pillow can make hemorrhoids worse! When your buttocks sink down into the hole, pressure is placed on the anal veins, causing more pain and inflammation. Instead, use a regular pillow for comfort so that weight is distributed and not placed on the veins.

244.   Cypress oil has been known for its healing properties for years. Applied to painful, inflamed hemorrhoids, it can bring some relief to those who suffer! Cypress oil can be found in health food stores and you can also buy it online. While it may not cure hemorrhoids, a little relief can put a smile back on your face!

245.   Never rush your bathroom time. Give yourself plenty of time to use the toilet, as the faster you rush, the harder you will push. Pushing can cause massive pain, swelling, and irritation of your hemorrhoids. Causing the least amount of pressure possible is the best way to relieve yourself of this painful situation.

246.   If you are looking for quick relief of a hemorrhoid flare up, you should check out some of the over-the-counter products available for just that purpose. There are creams, suppositories, gels and pads that contain medicines that numb the area. Other medicines such as Tylenol and Advil can help to reduce the pain as well.

247.   Don't be embarrassed to discuss your hemorrhoid problems with your doctor. By age 50, about half of all Americans will have suffered from hemorrhoids at one time or another. It's a common problem that your doctor has seen before, and it can be very uncomfortable, so don't be afraid to ask for the treatment you need.

248.   Your diet can have a significant impact on whether or not you are more prone to suffering from hemorrhoids. Certain foods and drinks can be especially irritating as they pass through the bowels. A diet that is filled with overly spicy foods or strong beverages like coffee, soda, and alcohol will put you at greater risk of forming hemorrhoids.

249.   If you are presently suffering from either internal or external hemorrhoids, you should avoid wiping with ordinary dry toilet paper. Instead, use a moistened bathroom towelette that contains aloe vera, or use a medicated wipe. Dry toilet paper can

leave residue; it can also aggravate the sensitive, inflamed tissues of the hemorrhoid.

250.   If you are prone to hemorrhoids and you have a job that requires a lot of sitting, then you need to get up and move a few minutes each hour. Exercise is very important in the prevention and treatment of hemorrhoids. Also, you will want to refrain from heavy lifting and anal intercourse to avoid the risk of developing hemorrhoids.

251.   When you are at the gym, refrain from lifting weights that are too strenuous. As you lift heavy weights, the muscles in your groin will contract, which can irritate and worsen your hemorrhoids. Try not to implement any body building exercises at the gym when you are affected with this condition.

252.   Though laxatives can temporarily relieve constipation, they are not a good solution for frequent hemorrhoids. Laxatives are meant to be a temporary solution to constipation, not hemorrhoids. If you are having trouble with bowel movements, consider making diet changes to even things out.

253.   To avoid getting hemorrhoids don't just sit there and worry about it and read about it constantly. Get up and go do something about it. The positive

attitude and movement of not sitting around all the time will increase health in your body, which decreases your chances of getting hemorrhoids. So if you get up to do something about hemorrhoids, it's a double-whammy. It may sound redundant and even ridiculous, but if you think it through, you see that it works.

254.   Nine out of ten times, hemorrhoids are to blame. However, you may wish to verify this with your physician. Rectal bleeding or blood in your stool could also be warning signs of something far more severe, like cancer. You will rest easier knowing exactly what the source of the problem is. If the diagnosis is hemorrhoids, your physician can provide you with an effective treatment plan.

255.   Many people like to read while sitting on the toilet. This is a perfect way to get hemorrhoids. You can be sitting much longer than you need to be, and pushing a little harder without even realizing it. If you are sitting longer than 5 minutes without anything happening, you have been sitting too long.

256.   Try adding more high fiber foods to your diet. More fiber translates into softer stools. Softer stools let you use less force when going to the bathroom, and will help minimize any pain or discomfort you may feel when pushing. Including raw fruits and

vegetables in your daily diet will serve you well, as will taking a daily fiber supplement.

257.   Always use a moist wipe. Wiping with dry paper can irritate and tear your hemorrhoids, so always use wet tissue paper, a moist wipe, or running water to clean and soothe yourself. If you wipe with dry tissue and see blood, you should immediately move to a moistened wipe of some sort.

258.   You should consult a medical professional if you experience prolonged or excessive bleeding from hemorrhoids. In rare cases excessive blood loss from hemorrhoids has caused anemia and alternative treatments like surgery or rubber band ligation may be required to treat hemorrhoids. It is also possible that the bleeding indicates a more serious condition that needs immediate medical attention.

259.   If you are having a painful hemorrhoid flare-up, a donut cushion may provide you with some relief. This donut cushion is specially designed to provide you with the most comfort as you deal with hemorrhoids. You will find that sitting on this type of cushion is far more comfortable than sitting on a hard surface.

260.   Eat plenty of garlic. Garlic has been shown to help soothe the intestines, which in turn helps to relieve swelling and pain associated with hemorrhoids. Most doctors recommend eating at least 2 full cloves a day for the maximum benefits, and some doctors even say you can insert a clove in the rectum.

261.   Sitting for long periods at work can increase the irritating symptoms of hemorrhoids. Be sure to get up and walk around frequently to relieve pressure. And remember to avoid activities that can worsen your symptoms, such as sitting too long on the toilet and heavy lifting.

262.   If you want to avoid the instances of hemorrhoids, then you need to be sure you get enough fiber in your diet. If you are finding this difficult through diet alone, you can try the various fiber supplements available without a prescription from the pharmacy or grocery store. Your aim is to get 20 to 35 grams per day.

263.   If you are presently suffering from either internal or external hemorrhoids, you should avoid wiping with ordinary dry toilet paper. Instead, use a moistened bathroom towelette that contains aloe vera, or use a medicated wipe. Dry toilet paper can

leave residue; it can also aggravate the sensitive, inflamed tissues of the hemorrhoid.

264.   If you are in a lot of pain from your hemorrhoids, go into your freezer and make an ice pack to put on your skin. Ice can help to numb the irritating aspects of your hemorrhoids, and can provide temporary relief for your skin. Apply ice to your skin for a quick solution.

265.   Keep your anal area as clean as possible. You should take the time to clean the area several times a day so that you can avoid getting the hemorrhoids infected. The anal area is prone to bacterial infections, and if you are not careful to keep it clean, the infections can lead to abscesses in the area.

266.   Don't depend on medications. Stimulant laxative drugs such as Bisacodyl tablets are meant to be used on a short-term basis and will not cure constipation. They may help with one bowel movement, but you'll be more constipated later. Side effects may include upset stomach, diarrhea, stomach cramps, faintness and stomach & intestinal irritation.

267.   If you don't get enough fruit and vegetables in your regular diet, it is important to take a daily fiber supplement. These supplements should be spread

out during the day, and you need to make sure you drink plenty of water.

268.   You should drink eight eight-ounce glasses of water each day to help you to prevent hemorrhoids. Also, water is needed to soften your stool which will also reduce the pain related to hemorrhoids. Limiting alcohol and caffeine intake can also work in your favor, as they both promote loss of water from your body. Keep yourself hydrated, drink enough water.

269.   Maintaining adequate hydration is essential when you suffer with hemorrhoids. This tip will help avoid the pain and discomfort of hemorrhoids. Water is a wonderful remedy for constipation, which is a common cause of hemorrhoids. This is also a good way to remove toxins from your body. Drink ten glasses a day, or more.

270.   Stay clean! Take care of your hemorrhoids! When you go to the restroom, make sure you clean the area thoroughly, taking care not to irritate it. If your bottom is not clean, bacteria can make its way into your hemorrhoids, and cause inflammation or even an abscess. To prevent these painful occurrences, make sure you wash well and prevent irritation!

271.   To help clear up your hemorrhoids, the first step is to relieve the symptoms. Constipation is a common cause of hemorrhoids, so make sure that your diet is healthy and rich in fiber. Eat lots of fruits and vegetables. Keep the anal area clean to help reduce the painful swelling and itching.

272.   Hemorrhoids can start to really itch and burn, but one of the last things you should ever do is scratch at them. It's very tempting to reach up there and alleviate that immediate itching sensation, but doing this will cause discomfort and possibly even pain for hours on end or until you apply some medication.

273.   After getting out of the bath or shower, try to avoid drying your rectum with a towel if you hope to avoid any hemorrhoid pain associated with flare-ups. Instead, opt for air-drying the area. This may take a little while longer, but you will most definitely appreciate the results here.

274.   When it comes to the many tips you'll read in your lifetime, you'll find that a lot of them have to do with water in some form or another, and it's no different with this hemorrhoid tip. If you want to help out your hemorrhoid, drink a lot of water to keep your digestive tract lubricated and your stools moving along nicely.

275.   Stay away from spicy and hot foods because they can inflame your hemorrhoids. Just making a few small changes in your diet can help you treat your current difficulties and help you prevent further complications. It is also important to limit the amount of coffee and beer that you drink.

276.   A great tip for your painful hemorrhoids is to avoid using regular toilet tissue. This is important because the friction of even soft tissue will only aggravate your hemorrhoid and cause more pain. Try using baby wipes or any other pre-treated wipe that will not cause too much friction.

277.   A great tip for your painful hemorrhoids is to try using some of the popular ointments or creams meant specifically for this purpose. There is a reason why these exist and they do tend to work for many people. Give it a try, just be sure to not over do it.

278.   A great tip for your painful hemorrhoids is to consider seeing a doctor if you notice any extreme increase in pain. This is important because it could be a symptom of something worse that might require surgery. Your doctor is a professional and it will be less embarrassing than you imagine.

279.   Constipation can contribute to the development of hemorrhoids or make them worse if you currently have them. Consume a diet rich in high-fiber foods or take a fiber supplement every day. Drink plenty of water along with the extra fiber as this will help your stool to become softer and easier to pass.

280.   If you prefer more natural ingredients for treating your ailments, consider purchasing a salve, ointment, or cream that contains horse chestnut. This botanical product, which is very popular in European countries, can be applied directly to external hemorrhoids. Within minutes, the topical solution will shrink the size of the hemorrhoid and offer relief from stinging sensations.

281.   Consider the usage of witch hazel for relief from hemorrhoid discomforts. It has astringent qualities able to reduce the size of, and cut blood flow to the hemorrhoid, prompting healing to begin. You can easily apply a cotton ball or pad soaked in witch hazel to the affected area for 5 minutes. A few drops in a sitz bath may also help.

282.   If you suffer from hemorrhoids, prevent further aggravation of the condition by keeping substances that contain scents, dyes, and essential oils away from the inflamed area. Even brief contact with

these ingredients may cause sharp pain, burning and inflammation.

283.   While treating your hemorrhoids, it is best to keep the anal area as dry as possible throughout the day to reduce the risk of additional irritation or infection of the tissues. Absorb excess moisture by applying a small amount of cornstarch or fragrance-free baby powder to your anal area once or twice per day.

284.   If you are prone hemorrhoids you may want to look into your daily routine. If you find yourself during to often then try to reduce the time periods during which you are sitting. Excessive sitting is a we ok known cause for hemorrhoids. If sitting can't be avoided take standing breaks.

285.   There are two types of hemorrhoids that are common in humans and while they have many similarities there are also several key differences. The most common and easiest type of this is an external hemorrhoid which is really not all that different from a varicose vein and can be treated very easily.

286.   One of the things that you will need to be aware of with hemorrhoids is the impact of coughing. Try to refrain from coughing as much as possible, since

this motion can strain the area of your body that is affected. Take medication if you are not able to control your cough.

287.   Avoid straining when you are using the bathroom. If you are pushing really hard to complete your mission, it is best to just stop and go for a walk until you feel the urge again. Straining will cause hemorrhoids to form, and you will be very uncomfortable for a long time.

288.   To relieve the pain, itching and inflammation of hemorrhoids, try medicated witch hazel pads. These special pads are soaked in witch hazel and can be tucked against the hemorrhoid to soothe the irritated area while shrinking the swelling. Witch hazel towelettes are also available, if you prefer a swipe-and-go solution.

289.   Alternate sitting and standing. Staying in either position for too long can actually irritate your hemorrhoids. If you stand or sit for too long, pressure begins to build on them, causing increased pain the next time you attempt to defecate. Try to only stay in one position for an hour at most.

290.   Stay clean! Take care of your hemorrhoids! When you go to the restroom, make sure you clean the area thoroughly, taking care not to irritate it. If

your bottom is not clean, bacteria can make its way into your hemorrhoids, and cause inflammation or even an abscess. To prevent these painful occurrences, make sure you wash well and prevent irritation!

291.   If you are having a painful hemorrhoid flare-up, a donut cushion may provide you with some relief. This type of cushion is designed for your bottom to provide you with optimum comfort while sitting during a breakout of hemorrhoids. Just sit down on one, and you'll feel much more at ease than you would sitting on most anything else.

292.   Hemorrhoids flare up on us the most when we have trouble passing a stool. This means you should always work to have looser stools by way of a stool softener. You can get some great over-the-counter products that will keep things moving along nicely down there, allowing you to use the bathroom comfortably.

293.   Overweight individuals are at a bigger risk for hemorrhoids, so you should lose weight if you want to reduce your risk or reduce the swelling of a pre-existing hemorrhoid. A larger waist and abdominal area means that you are putting g a lot more weight on the veins in your rectum.

294.   If you cannot find any special type of toilet paper out there that's easier on your anus, you should try making sure you only wipe your rear with toilet paper that is wet. This will certainly help to eliminate the friction and create a softer barrier between the paper and the swollen veins in your rectum.

295.   Keep it as clean as possible. If your hemorrhoid breaks open and bleeds, and then becomes dirty, it could get infected. You could eventually get an abscess in the are, requiring medical attention or surgery. Use a damp, clean cloth to gently clean the area when you bathe, so as not to inflame it.

296.   While many people feel that hemorrhoids are very embarrassing, this affliction is very common. If you notice blood or believe that you may be suffering from hemorrhoids in conjunction with a blood clot, it is imperative that you make an appointment with your doctor. The faster you seek help, the faster you can be done with the ordeal.

297.   If you have hemorrhoids and find that your problem hasn't taken care of itself after a couple of weeks or the problem seems to be getting worse quickly than you should go to a professional immediately. Probably you will have no major

problems but they will be able to tell you exactly what is going on.

298.   When you are affected with hemorrhoids, avoid drinking hot coffee or eating hot soup. Hot foods can irritate the surface of your skin and will increase the pain that you feel during the night. Stick to sandwiches, fruit and vegetables to optimize the way that you feel during your meals.

299.   In the morning, one of the best drinks that you can have is vegetable juice for your hemorrhoids. Vegetable juice will give you the nutrients that you need to improve blood circulation in your body and can reduce your level of toxins. Drink 16-20 ounces of vegetable juice to start your morning off right.

300.   Exercise caution when using medicines that relieve constipation. While these laxative products can help you in the short term, you can quite easily experience constipation after the effects have worn off. Many times the constipation is worse than you started with. Look for natural ways to soften your stool or seek a physician's advice.

301.   To stay as healthy as possible and limit the symptoms of hemorrhoids, make sure that you maintain a proper diet. This means that you should reduce the foods that have high cholesterol and fat

content to improve the way that you feel. Eat well-balanced meals that are rich in protein for optimal results.

302.   To reduce the chances of developing hemorrhoids, maintain a healthy weight. Being overweight puts excessive pressure on the pelvic region and the pelvic veins. The best way to maintain a healthy weight and prevent hemorrhoids, is to get plenty of exercise and eat a well balanced diet that is high in fiber.

303.   Alternate sitting and standing. Staying in either position for too long can actually irritate your hemorrhoids. If you stand or sit for too long, pressure begins to build on them, causing increased pain the next time you attempt to defecate. Try to only stay in one position for an hour at most.

304.   Use a hemorrhoid cream sparingly. The use of cream will only reduce the pain, it will not take away any swelling you are experiencing. If you plan on using the cream beyond seven days, seek medical advice from your physician first. Applying them too frequently can actually result in greater discomfort.

305.   Hemorrhoids are a common and irritating complication of pregnancy. It's important to avoid any natural or over-the-counter remedies until you

consult with your doctor to see what is safe for you and your baby. Try sleeping on your left side to reduce pressure on certain veins that can make hemorrhoids swell.

306.   Sitting for long periods at work can increase the irritating symptoms of hemorrhoids. Be sure to get up and walk around frequently to relieve pressure. And remember to avoid activities that can worsen your symptoms, such as sitting too long on the toilet and heavy lifting.

307.   Hemorrhoids can start to really itch and burn, but one of the last things you should ever do is scratch at them. It's very tempting to reach up there and alleviate that immediate itching sensation, but doing this will cause discomfort and possibly even pain for hours on end or until you apply some medication.

308.   To avoid flare ups of hemorrhoid symptoms and facilitate your movement, try squatting over the toilet instead of sitting. This position, while awkward, can eliminate some of the pain associated with your bowel movement and make it more comfortable.

309.   Many people suffer from the painful, embarrassing symptoms of hemorrhoids. One

home remedy that can help is garlic! Garlic has been used for many medical problems for years. Try ingesting 2 garlic cloves 2-3 times per day to relieve hemorrhoids that are painful or bleeding. You can also insert a clove of garlic inside the anus to feel the healing effects.

310.   Hemorrhoids can have many irritating and painful symptoms. These include pain, itching, inflammation and bleeding. For some quick relief, a good home remedy is apple cider vinegar. Dip a cotton swab in the vinegar and dab it gently over the inflamed hemorrhoids. Do this twice a day for soothing relief.

311.   If you experience diarrhea on more than three to four bowel movements, it's time to schedule an appointment with your doctor. Chronic diarrhea will irritate your bowels, and can cause hemorrhoids to enlarge greatly and possibly tear. Prevent this by eating fiber and staying well hydrated.

312.   To reduce the symptoms that you have from hemorrhoids, apply a thin layer of aloe gel to the affected area of your skin. Aloe gel will help to reduce the inflammation that you have, by creating a rich layer of protection so that air does not irritate your skin surface.

313.   If you have a very firm chair at work, bring a cushion to sit on during the day. This cushion can reduce the amount of friction that you have on your skin, which can limit the sores that you acquire. Find a soft gel cushion to sit on while at work.

314.   If you suffer from hemorrhoids, try taking an iron supplement if you do not have much iron in your diet. The iron will soften your stools, making them less painful to pass. Take the supplements all throughout the day, and don't forget to drink your eight glasses of water.

315.   Try using an ice pack to reduce swelling and alleviate pain from a hemorrhoid flareup. Some people also find applying over the counter creams or witch hazel to the affected area helpful in reducing swelling. To prevent further hemorrhoid irritation use a donut pillow when sitting or avoid sitting altogether.

316.   If you have been having chronic hemorrhoid pain and it does not seem to ever get better, see your doctor. There are surgical procedures that are very safe and simple that can help with hemorrhoids.

317.   It is a good idea to go to your doctor and have the area checked out. The blood you see on your

toilet paper or in your stool might be from a more serious condition.

318.   The most effective way to prevent hemorrhoids is to make sure your stool is not hard. Having to push out hard stools will irritate your anus, and ultimately, cause hemorrhoids. Try to eat foods that contain a lot of fiber, such as vegetables, and purchase a stool softener if needed.

319.   If you have hemorrhoids and you are in excruciating pain, see your doctor immediately. This could be a sign of a thrombosed hemorrhoid, which is a blood clot that forms inside the hemorrhoid. This should be treated immediately.

320.   Hemorrhoid cushions can be really expensive, a great alternative to use is a soft pillow. A pillow has more give to it than the air inside of the rubber casing for a cusion. The air in the pillow can escape and will allow the pillow to conform to your bottom, whereas the rubber air-filled cushion will not conform quite as well.

321.   Applying ointment directly to a hemorrhoid is a good way to help shrink the size of it. A hemorrhoid is a swollen, possibly ruptured vein, so a medicine like Neosporin can help to heal the sore

partially. It will not completely remove the hemorrhoid, but it will help in reducing the size.

322.   Don't expect laxatives or stool softeners to fix a hemorrhoid. Laxatives are not a long-term solution to the constipation issue that brought about the hemorrhoid in the first place. Also, while a laxative may make the passing of stool easier, it doesn't actually fix the hemorrhoid. It simply reduces the symptoms.

323.   Overweight individuals are at a bigger risk for hemorrhoids, so you should lose weight if you want to reduce your risk or reduce the swelling of a pre-existing hemorrhoid. A larger waist and abdominal area means that you are putting g a lot more weight on the veins in your rectum.

324.   The swollen veins and resulting pain that accompany hemorrhoids is believed to benefit from consuming vitamin A. Try eating more carrots or drinking carrot juice to get a good boost of vitamin A to help your hemorrhoids.

325.   As far as products go, there are plenty of treatments that you can choose from when it comes to your hemorrhoids and one of the best is a numbing topical spray that you can purchase. This spray is easy to apply and works to numb the pain.

It won't really help it to heal, but it will numb the pain.

326.   When you use the restroom, do not push too hard. This will exacerbate your hemorrhoids; instead, try walking around to see if it makes you feel like using the bathroom. If that does not work, try engaging in light exercise to get your bowels moving. No matter what, do not force yourself.

327.   Are you looking for natural ways to alleviate the pain, itching and swelling of hemorrhoids? Here is a tip that may help! For pain and swelling, aloe vera can offer quick relief. You can try an aloe vera gel, or if you have access to an aloe vera plant, take the outer layer off of a leaf and place the leaf around the anal area. This technique can soothe pain and itching as well as inflammation!

328.   Those affected by painful hemorrhoids may be able to find relief by using topical medications intended to alleviate the sensations of burning that can sometimes occur. By using this type of treatment, it is possible to reduce inflammation, limit swelling and eradicate pain. However, it is important to realize that the relief provided may only be temporary in nature.

329.   If you find yourself suffering from hemorrhoids be sure to wear 100% cotton underwear. This will allow the area to breathe, which will reduce the healing time, and will also be less irritating if it comes into contact with the area than the other types of material underwear often is made of.